Do You Know Lisa?
Collection of Health Questions, Answers, and Tips. Volume 3

Dr. Lisa Goins PhD, APRN, FNP-BC, RMT

Welcome to Volume 3 of *Do You Know Lisa?*

Have you ever wanted to ask a provider a question about a health problem, idea, or holistic intervention but was too shy or not sure they would answer you? Sometimes there is a go to person that folks know and will sent you to, if you should ask them.

But where did the title of this book come from? A few years back, Lisa was boarding a late flight out of CVG airport to go the National Association of Nurse Practitioners Convention. A lot of Nurse Practitioners were taking this late flight after working all day. Everyone was boarding when it was Lisa's turn to board the plane. Nurse Practitioners began saying "Hey! It is Lisa!" A big meet and greet began, as everyone introduced themselves until the others on the plane were beginning to wonder who this person was. This flight just happened to have two well-known Cincinnati baseball players on board, when one of the players leaned over to the other and asked "Do you know Lisa?" The other baseball player looked up at the Nurse Practitioner, smiled and nodded. "Hi Pete!" Said Lisa.

Do you know Lisa? She can answer those questions or find out the answers for you. This book is a collection of questions, answers, tips published on many social media sites for the year 2016. You can follow or submit questions to Lisa's health articles on the internet at www.couturehealthcare.org.

After all, you do know Lisa!

Who is this Lisa you speak about?

About the Author: Lisa Goins PhD, APRN, FNP-BC, RMT is the CEO and Founder of Couture Health Care. Dr. Goins started out in nursing as a resident care tech, LPN, RN, RN-ASN, RN-BSN, RN-MSN, and RN-DNPc. Dr. Goins is a Board Certified Family Nurse Practitioner in the State of Ohio. Dr. Goins then completed a non-secular Bachelors, Masters, and PhD. Dr. Goins holds a clergy licenses in the State of Ohio and is a Reiki Master/Teacher.

Dr. Goins' health articles feature a mix of holistic health, wealth, spiritual, and information for health professionals and the public. Dr. Goins' health articles and videos may be found on Google+, Twitter, LinkedIn, Facebook, YouTube, and CoutureHealthCare.org.
Dr. Goins sees patients at Couture Health Care, 201 North Brookwood Ave., Hamilton, OH, 45013. Office number: 513-857-5679.

Couture Health Care is an IRS recognized 501c3 Corporation that started out with house calls in Ohio and began offering office visits in October 2015. Services offered include Nurse Practitioner visits for primary health care, spiritual and counseling, and reiki.

In addition to working with Couture Health Care, Dr. Goins also works with companies Dwarven Tavern and Foundation for Spiritual Research.

Dr. Goins is the author of the following books, which may be found on Lulu and Amazon for purchase.

Dragon Prophecy- Published (Fantasy) December 27, 2009

Do You Know Lisa? 2014 Collection of Health Questions, Answers, and Tips. – Published (Health Care) December 26, 2014

Dwarven Tavern Story Hooks: Quick Start Story Ideas- Published (Fantasy) December 23, 2014

CEO Business Objectives: Health, Wealth, and Success- Published (Business) April 3, 2015

Do You Know Lisa? Collection of Health Questions, Answers, and Tips. Book 2. – Published (Health Care) October 25, 2015

Do You Know Lisa? Collection of Health Questions, Answers, and Tips. Volume 3 – Published (Health Care) November 2016

Dedication:
Thank you to all the donors, sponsors, fans, supporters, and patients of Couture Health Care.

Special thanks to Couture Health Care's staff for helping make the impossible, possible every day for our patients.

Ultimate thanks to Couture Health Care's Board Members in believing in me and reminding me I can do this.

Disclaimer:
This collection of works is not a replacement for visiting your Nurse Practitioner. Standards of Care updated periodically, therefore it is recommended to visit your Nurse Practitioner for your health care needs at least yearly. After all, Dr. Lisa always tells her patients that the last words with *Dr. Google* is you may have cancer. Not everyone has cancer, but if you do, your Nurse Practitioner can help get you the care you need. Many health articles are written in generalization and may not be written by health care providers online but those with writing degrees. Dr. Goins recommends that seeing your Nurse Practitioner provider will help *couture* your health care for you.

Information:
The information gathered here in the following writings may change with new standards of care, implemented technology in the health care world, and if the material OFFENDS thee, put the book down or give it away to someone else.

Editing:
Typos and errors can happen and do. My apologies in advance. Dr. Lisa also views typos and errors as copy rights. Win-win.

Thank you for purchasing in print or downloading this book to read. I appreciate your support and may you find the content information useful in your daily life. Please follow up with a review after your reading online and do share the book with friends and family. Blessings! May your health be excellent…if not, give me or your local Nurse Practitioner a call.

"Ideas are easy. It is implementing them that is the hard part."

~Dr. Lisa Goins PhD, APRN, FNP-BC, RMT

Contents:

Nurse Practitioner Visit:

What is a Nurse Practitioner?   11

Facebook vs. Medical Provider   13

Appointment Time Starts Now!   14

What is a Welcome Visit?   15

What is a Follow Up Visit?   16

What is a Flat Rate?   17

Please Fill This Out   18

Multiple Providers in One Office   19

Transportation Struggles for Patients   20

Debt:

Debt Free with Health Prevention   21

Debt Free with Better Immunity   22

Insurance:

Welcome to the World of Health Insurance   23

Two Insurances Instead of One.   24

My Insurance Was Bought By Another!   25

Insurance Changes Provider Will Not See Me!   26

Self-Pay Vs Insurance   31

Pre-Authorizations for Medications   32

Medication Discount Cards   33

Patients Get Insurance Books   34

Insurance Deductibles Come First   35

Paying Insurance Co-Payments   36

Write Off Insurance Paid Bills   37

Ten Percent Donation   38

Health Care Savings:

Health Care Savings with Health Care Accounts   39

Health Care Savings with Health Maintenance   40

Health Care Savings with Cash   41

Health Care Savings with Insurance   42

Health Care Savings with a Medicine Closet   43

Dyslexia:

Dyslexia and Test Taking   44

Dyslexia and Sleep   46

Dyslexia and Colors   47

Dyslexia and Chunking.   48

Dyslexia and Your Other Left   51

Quitting Smoking:

Quitting Smoking with a New Habit   52

Quitting Smoking with Medications   53

Quitting Smoking with Others   54

Quitting Smoking by Removing One   55

Quit Smoking by Smoking   56

Prepare to be an Ex-Smoker   57

Smoke Less in a Month   58

Three Ways to Quit Smoking   59

Depression:

Depression and Vitamin D3   60

Depression Risk for Suicide.   61

Depression Signs and Symptoms   62

Depression   63

First Responders:

First Responders Preparations   64

First Responders Emotions   65

First Responders to Public Shooting Events   66

First Responder for Shot Gun Wounds   67

Summer Time:

Summer Time Shut In   68

Summer Time Bone Health   69

Summer Time FREE Vitamin D   70

Want Fabulous Hair?   71

Summer Time Vitamins   72

Holiday:

Annual Mother's Day Pass It forward   73

Forever Christmas   74

Breakfast:

Breakfast is Important   75

Diet:

500 Calorie Give Away Diet Plan   76

Weight Loss By Counting Calories   77

Military:

Boots and Siblings   80

Boots and Boxes   81

Boots in House   82

Vaccines:

Baby Shower Vaccines   83

Adult Child Goes Against Parent's Decision   84

Pets

Rehome the Family Pets   85

Questions for Dr. Lisa

Three reasons life is on your nerves.   86

Six ways to get cheaper medications.   87

Should I keep taking diabetic medication?   88

Heart

Fast Pumping, Go!   89

Three Fast Heart Facts!   90

Hard Restart

Hard Restart- Strength to Weaknesses   91

Hard Restart Deteriorating Health   92

Hard Restart Tiny X of Life   93

Hard Restart-Emoticons of Feelings   94

Hard Life Restart-The Basics   95

Winter:

Wicking Cold!   96

Freezing? Do Housework!   97

What is a Nurse Practitioner?

A patient wanted to know what a Nurse Practitioner is and how are they different from other nurses?

First we show you the order on how nurses progress with degrees and licenses. This is not a complete list but gives the reader an idea what types of nursing there is.

- Health care personnel. These are unlicensed staff members who care for patients in their homes, provide company, and help get them to activities. This person is not a nurse.

- Medical Assistant (MA). This is a person that is trained and holds a certification or a two year degree. This person works under the supervision of any type of nurse. This person can do office paperwork, give shots under supervision, and may have clinical training per classes or grandfathered since they were by trained providers. This person is not a nurse but a technician.

- State Certified Nursing Assistants (STNA), Certified Nursing Assistants (CNA) or nursing assistants. Staff members that do personal care, such as baths, helping patients dress, and helping them eat. STNAs hold a certification with training. No licenses. Work under the supervision of a Licensed Practical Nurse (LPN) or Registered Nurse (RN). This person is not a nurse.

- Licensed Practical Nurse (LPN). Is a nurse with one year to two years of education and a state licenses to practice. LPNs can pass medications, do vital signs, take orders, and call providers for orders. Additional training in some states allows LPNs to do IV fluids and manage IV lines. LPNs work under the supervision of a Registered Nurse (RN).

- Registered Nurse (RN-ASN). Is a nurse with either two years of education and licenses called an Associate Registered Nurse. STNAs and LPNs work under their supervision. RNs can administer all types of meds, blood products, and jobs range from ICU to management positions.

- Registered Nurses (RN-BSN). Is a nurse with four years of education, one or two degrees (ASN and BSN or just BSN). RNs types make work together but the RN BSN will be the nurse who is the in charge for a unit, building or also known as Director of Nursing (DON) or Assistant Director of Nursing (ADON).

- Masters in Nursing (MSN). This nurse may hold several degrees before getting their masters. Nurses at this level are also referred as Advanced Practice Nurses (APN) or Advanced Practice Registered Nurses (APRN). APRNs are Midwives (bring babies in the world), Clinical Specialist (Advanced care and treatments), and Nurse Practitioners (Primary Care Providers). All will hold several degree, RN and APN licenses, and board certifications in order to practice in their specialty. APRNs are also referred to as general primary care providers. APRNs can order medications, treatments, do referrals, and own their own companies that provide health care.

- Doctor of Nursing (DNP) or PhD. This nurse holds an additional degree that is called a terminal degree. This is as highest degree a nurse can hold. This allows the nurse to be called doctor. This degree does not have a licenses at this time. There is a board certification that may be taken if wished but not required at this time.

  So a nurse isn't just a nurse.

Facebook vs. Medical Provider

Many parents will turn to Facebook to complain or look for advice. This many include current medical treatments received from a medical provider. That may be fine and acceptable, to want to vent or wonder, if the medical advice is the standard or if there might be other options.

But what is not acceptable is when a parent release medical history and details to the public. This may be a violating the child's rights and may be a violation of the Health Insurance Portability and Accountability Act (HIPAA). Remember, Facebook and all such systems, saves all content on long term hard storage servers. The information will be there for decades. This may be damaging to a child later on in their life.

What makes this look even worse is when the parent wishes to be non-complaint by not following through with said medical assessment, diagnosis, plan, and treatment. Again, there is a parent's choice but adverse reactions to the child, may result in legal issues later depending on the parent's non-compliance of the course of treatment and outcomes.

Thus, when it sounds as if you are asking for medical advice from a particular group, which is a Facebook group, not a medical group then parents may be violating their family/child's privacy by releasing health information. However, that is always a choice. The parent's non-compliance to follow their child's therapy based on non-medical advice on Facebook post verses their medical providers' advice, raises a lot of questions. Parents may wish to consider withdrawing their posts and avoid substituting non-health care providers for licensed medical professionals when deciding what is best for their child.

Should you not agree with the treatment, speak with the provider at the time of treatment and/or seek a second opinion of another licensed medical provider. Remember, the end goal is to protect and provide accurate/researched based health care to the child.

Appointment Time Starts Now!

Question: When does my appointment start?
Answer: The schedule time of your appointment begins at the time stated. If your appointment starts at 2 pm, it is 2 pm.

Why? The appointment time is with the provider. If you are late, the time is already ticking. If you need to fill out paperwork, then you need to do this first. If you need to show your ID and insurance cards, then this needs to be done before the appointment. If there are any papers that need to be filled out, then this needs to be done so the information can be entered into the computer or data base.

This may be followed by a short meeting with an assistant who will take your vital signs and list any medications into the computer or data base. Then you will be escorted to a room to see the provider. Or the provider will take this information should there not be an assistant.

Solution? Show up 15 minutes early to get any paperwork completed, forms filled out, ID and insurance information exchange completed. This helps cut out wait time for seeing the provider.

Delays: Computers and data bases can become bogged down with lots of users and if the machine gets hot. Patients can also cause delays be not being ready or prepared for the visit. Did you bring your list or bottles of medicine? Do you need to remove several layers of clothes to find your arm to place a blood pressure cuff? Patients with list of requests and just one more questions, can cause a thoughtful provider to run behind. If you need longer for an appointment, request the time. You may be asked to keep your questions limited to the top two or three major problems and reschedule for a lengthy list of questions.

Waiting? You may not be waiting on the provider, the provider may be waiting on you.

What is a Welcome Visit?

A welcome visit is your first visit at a provider's office. What is covered during this visit?

- Patient identification will be confirmed and the patient chart will be started.

- Office policies and procedures will be explained to you.

- Baseline vital signs will be taken.

- Health history that includes any surgeries, accidents, and if any health problem runs in the family.

- Medications. This is when you want to bring your list or bottles of medications to be checked and reviewed.

- Any prior health records, vaccinations, or other important information.

- A care plan will be started. This is an agreement between you and your provider on how you wish to move forward with health care objectives and goals.

The provider may change medications to meet the patient's needs better during this visit, order testing, laboratory work to be done in office or off site at another time.

Any additional information or education will be done at this visit or set up for another time to be completed.

Patients should leave with their next appointment scheduled with any follow up information addressed.

What is a Follow Up Visit?

Patients do not always understand why they need to return to see a provider. Providers follow rules, guidelines, and standards of care for prescribing and treating patients. This means that patients will need to be seen more than once in a year to get medications or treatments completed.

This allows providers to follow up on care patients have received. Providers can review with patients if medications are effective or need changed. If blood work interventions need to be done, such as starting a medication if cholesterol is too high. Patients may even need to be referred to a specialist and this is when the provider can give more education on how the process will work.

Follow up times will vary per provider or needs per patients based on the care needed.

What is a Flat Rate?

Sometimes a provider may charge what is called a flat rate. A flat rate includes the entire visit any prescriptions written at the time of visit.

Any laboratory work done at the office may be included or not in the cost. It will depend on the office's flat rate information.
Flat rates are for patients that have lost their insurance or do not have insurance and need care.

Flat rates are cheaper than insurance plans for patients that need health care when other options are not available to them.

Please Fill This Out.

Many times patients will present with papers to fill out and expect the paperwork to be completed when present. Many times the paperwork presented cannot be.
Patients need to be aware

- Paperwork needs time to be filled out.

- Finished paperwork will need to be picked up later.

- Additional charges for paperwork to complete by a provider may be in addition to visit.

- Last minute deadlines may not be met.

Ways to expedite your paperwork

- Complete all the necessary information.

- Sign, date, and provide identification when necessary

- Understand what part of the forms the provider needs to fill out.

- Understand any regulations for the requirement of paperwork and your duties on returning it.

Multiple Providers in One Office
It is not uncommon now days for many providers to work in the same offices with other providers. Providers may belong to the office or are contracted in to use services or office space to keep overhead low for the providers and increase convenience for patients.

This can become confusing for patients who are looking for one particular provider but cannot find them. It is the responsibility of the provider to give this additional information to patients.

Patients can help by

- Making sure they get the address and telephone number to get on spot directions if they get lost on the way.

- Ask what the building looks like and where to park or be dropped off.

- Ask where they may sit if their rides are running late.

- Bring something to read or keep themselves busy if waiting.

- Understand that waiting in an area for a ride may not be allowed due to limited seating for patients waiting for the provider.

Transportation Struggles for Patients

Transportation for health care visits can be a struggle when a patient does not have access to a car, bus services, and traveling by bicycle or walking is too far.

Money to pay for taxi or other services may be out of the question for those on strict incomes and budgets.
Another option is contacting your insurance company or provider to find out about transportation services in your area that you may qualify to receive.

Many Medicaid services are accepted by communities and companies willing to pick up patients and drive them to their appointments.

Prior to service needed, the patient will have to call 24-48 hours beforehand to set up appointment pick-ups.

Time to pick up for appointment and after appointment may leave gaps in additional waiting. This can be a problem if there is no place to wait or the office is very busy the day you visit.
To find out about services call your insurance company, human services/welfare department, and senior services or council on aging departments for more information.

You may also inquire at your provider's office to see which company is your local transportation option.

Debt Free with Health Prevention

Is it possible to be in debt to your health? Can debt be prevented by the individual with health prevention? Is this possible? Yes. It is. There are many ways to prevent getting sick and adding up additional cost to the budget. This can put an individual in the red very quickly.

One health prevention is getting a flu shot. How can this keep debt from incurring? Here are some ways debt does occur when an individual gets the flu.

⬜   Lost of work resulting in lost of wages. Average flu illness may have a person missing an entire week of pay approximately $200-$500 lost wages. Resulting in a rippling effect of debt growing. Resulting missed wages have to be made up and bills start falling behind. This can strain tight budgets.

⬜   When the primary care giver is sick, this results in everyone is home exposure to the illness or ill at the same time. There may be no one who can take care of the other or clean up after them. This includes helping to replace the primary care giver. Inability to clean, will keep germs lingering longer than they should in the home.

⬜   Additional needs for illness may not be in the budget. Cost for tissues, wipes, cleaning supplies, and foods/liquids to relieve symptoms.

So it is easy to see how an illness can ruin a budget and cause more debt.

Debt Free with Better Immunity

Becoming debt free is a goal for many folks. Debt often references owing money for something. What if we applied this to an individual's immunity? What if you could be in debt to your immunity? Is that possible?

An individual's immunity is what helps fight off illness and germs. An individual's immunity can be compromised in many ways. One way is to be too skinny or thin. Having a Body Mass Index (BMI) that is too low. A BMI is like square footage for the body. How tall against how much weight equals a number. A BMI too low, and there is not enough ingredients in the body to fuel the cells to fight off an illness.

Thus, if an individual gets sick, will they be able to recover? Is there enough fuel to help the cells in the body to kill off the invading germs? This can lead to a trip to a provider for medical care or a longer stay in the hospital because the body is fighting so hard to get better and it can't. Additional help is needed. This may result in medical bills that will add to not just the financial debt occurred but the debt to the body's immunity.

Welcome to the World of Health Insurance

Welcome to the world of health insurance. There are degrees of health insurance users.
Patients who:

- Were born with it, uses it regular, and never had a life without it.

- Had insurance with parents and find that out of the house equals out of insurance too.

- Have insurance through work with their jobs. Jobs change and so does insurance.

- Have between job insurance or fall on hard times, qualifies them for public assistance insurance.

- Never had insurance.

  Patients who have insurance now are stuck with finding a provider who will take the insurance they have. This may give the idea that some insurances are better than others.

  Nope, it just means that there are providers who have agreed to take the insurance based on the fact that insurance companies will pay providers in a timely fashion so the provider will stay in business. Insurances that likely to be late in paying, deny paying providers for work done, and fight over basic health care needs, may find that providers refuse to work with them. This leaves the patients with troubling insurance looking for new providers.

  Insurance may or may not be awesome for the patient. Patients may find their insurance has a high deductible, co-pays, and other limitations. This can limit insurance usage if a patient finds their life in a crisis. Health patients may find high deductibles work fine when they do not need crisis care.

  So having health insurance may be good or bad depending on who you speak with and how you use it.

Two Insurances Instead of One.

Instead of picking just once insurance policy, a person may have two or more. This can be a problem or a blessing. The blessing is when one insurance will not pay for the bill, the other insurance company will. It can be a problem when one insurance will not pay then the other figures it should not either. This can leave the patient responsible for the bill.

Another problem that results is when there is no clear who should be billed first. This problem results from the policy purchased or purchased for a dependent who may have additional insurance. A primary insurance needs to be chosen and when the bill is submitted for payment, that insurance should be billed first.

It is always good to know which insurance should be a primary and then a secondary. Other things to know is what each policy covers and what are the differences. It may cut a lot of red tape and make everyone happy if each insurance is billed for the services they have agreed to pay. It can help insure that the patient will not be left holding the bill.

My Insurance Was Bought By Another!

The last two years have been busy for insurance companies buying each other. This helps the insurance companies in several ways. It helps increase those insured and spreads the cost averaging over the entire group of patients. This can decrease cost for everyone and increase savings.

However, sometimes it can leave someone without insurance and thinking they have coverage. This can get very sticky for the person with the policy. Through no fault of their own, they have paid their policy, visited their provider, and kept up on everything they should have done.

To their surprise they receive a letter saying that the insurance company has been purchased and merged with another company.

The first things to do then will be:
Check the policy date of expiration.
Who should all the bills be forwarded to for payment or reimbursement?
Is the new company offering any changes in the policy?
What is the differences is the policy changes with the new company?

Notify your provider, if they have not notified you first. IF the company has closed the doors to accepting any bills, the policy holder/patient may now be responsible for the bill.

Rules and regulations do apply to all policies but payments to providers may be lost in the mess of changes. Being proactive can keep patients from having to pay more when it is unnecessary.

Insurance Changes Provider Will Not See Me!

A lot of thought goes into picking an insurance. Sometimes patients pick an insurance because they have established a relationship with a provider. This relationship is built on years of seeing a provider. The patient feels comfortable knowing their provider. The provider has met their needs and has typically rule out certain health problems or working on a care plan to keep health problems in check.

Here comes a wrench into a good working machine. The insurance changes and now the provider is no longer accepting the insurance. This leaves the patient with insurance but no provider. What happened?

Insurance companies will only accept so many providers in an area to contract with to take patients with their insurance and will agree to pay the provider an agreed fee. Sometimes an area will have too many providers accepting the insurance and decide to limit the providers. This can shut out providers and patients with insurance.

Insurance companies may sell or buy plans and condense their work force and contracts. This can also keep providers from accepting insurance from patients. New or old contracts are not options in the new company.

Providers who have trouble getting the insurance companies to pay for services provided to patients, may decide that after having insurance companies delaying payment for over three to six months, bouncing payment checks, or requiring too many pre-authorizations for routine medications thus adding more work for the same pay, becomes more work than worth taking.

Providers, like insurance companies do have to keep the lights on. Many providers may not keep the patients up to date on if their insurances are paying and may be surprise to get bills from companies not paying timely or find out their provider just cannot deal with the headache of trying to get an insurance to pay for services rendered months ago.

Then this leads to patients either switching insurances or providers.

How Does a Patient's Insurance Pay a Provider?

The patient arrives at the provider's office for care. The patient presents their insurance card. The insurance card is checked with the insurance company to see if it is still valid or active. If the insurance card is not active, then the patient will be notified that they no longer have insurance. Other arrangements to pay will be needed to set up at this time.

Next, the patient is seen and care provided. The provider charts or writes down the visit and what the patient's complaint was, what the provider saw, did, prescribed, and any testing ordered. The chart is coded for brevity and privacy by the provider and the provider's biller. This includes what the provider charged for care and this bill is sent to the insurance company to be paid by the insurance coverage.

The insurance company then gets this bill from the provider. The insurance company process lots of bills daily. The insurance company may not be working on current bills, so the bill will go in cue to be processed. This could be days or months before the bill is reviewed and a decision to pay or not.

If the bill is decided not to be paid, the bill will return to the provider for any corrections or the decision has been decided that the bill will never be paid due to lack of qualifications of insurance coverage or other such problem. The provider can then send this bill to the patient to be paid or back to the insurance company to be disputed to be paid.

et us hope your provider will fight to get it paid by your insurance. Again, the bill sent may or not be decided to be paid. This cycle of events may take up to six months or more to resolve. This is why patients think bills were paid at the time of visit, may then get a bill "out of the blue" from their provider to be paid. This may also cause patients to find they suddenly cannot be seen because they owe the provider for an old bill.

If the bill is decided to be paid, then the funds will be sent to the provider. The provider then notes that the care rendered was paid and the patient's account will be adjusted accordingly to show the changes.

In conclusion, insurance may pay quickly with turn-around of paying for the bill in days or months. The result may reflect on if your provider continues to take the insurance at their location. This can jeopardize patient-provider relationships when insurances change policies, payment plans, or insurance companies are purchased by another insurance company.

Need to Change Providers

Accepting a new insurance or changing insurance leads to finding a provider who will accept the insurance. After the insurance is picked, the insurance company has a list of provider the insurance company has contracted to accept their insurance policies.

The list of providers may be online and in a printed book that will be mailed out to the policy holder. Individuals may pick a provider for many reasons. Close to their home, available by public transportation, female or male, many providers or one provider at a location, or particular services offered, such as primary care or general practice.

Insurance companies typically wish for the individuals to pick a primary care provider first. This is the person who will help the individual to get referrals to other providers based on needs. Many providers may not accept patients without referrals and a referral may also be necessary to get the insurance company to pay for services.

Example, a primary care provider discovers a heart problem and refers a patient to a heart/cardiologist for follow up. A female patient may be expecting. She will need not only someone to deliver the baby/gynecologist/midwife but maybe a provider/pediatrician/specialist for the baby too.

To switch providers, is to find a new provider on the list of the insurance companies and check to see if the provider is taking new patients. Sometimes providers are seeing the maximum number of patients they can safely see in a day and stop taking new patients. If the provider is taking new patients, then showing up with identification, insurance card, any medication bottles of current prescription medications taken, and any old records will help get the individual established as a new patient. Old records typically need a signed released and are responsibility of the old provider's office and patient to be moved forward.

The new provider will review the records, medications, and may new changes in the health care plan for the patient. Always plan for the first visit to be the longest. It does take time to get everything set up so the next visit can be shorter.

Self-Pay Vs Insurance

Not everyone has insurance. This means that the individual is a self-pay and responsible for the bill that will be generated. If a patient is going to be self-pay, it is good to let the office know up front. This can keep cost down for the patient.

The patient may decline pain medication in the hospital or urgent care because the medication may be cheaper at the pharmacy. Patients may opt out of testing and decide to move testing to a later date if deemed medically necessary at the time. Patients may need to pay the bill up front or make other arrangements.

Patients may also use health care accounts to pay for bills. Health care accounts may be tax deferred dollars that will help keep the cost of money not budgeted for visits, in budget.

Health care accounts may also allow patients to manage their health care better by targeting a date when any and all testing can be done with payment. Thus, accounts with no roll over to the next year, that money will need to be spent. This is one way to help keep annual cost in check and annual testing compliant.

Pre-Authorizations for Medications

Insurances may not pay for medications or they may need what is called a pre-authorization. A pre-authorization is paperwork that needs to be filled out saying that other medications did not work or other information required by the insurance company before they will pay it.

Depending on the medication, the provider may have to speak with the insurance or pharmacy or both to state that another medication was tried and was not effective as the medication that was prescribed.

Pre-authorizations may deny medications not paid by the insurance for any reason. So even if a provider fills them out, the medication can still be denied.

However, free medications and paid for in cash medications do not need pre-authorizations. Not that everyone wants to pay hundreds of dollars for medication that their insurance company will pay for them to have, but it is an option.

Medication Discount Cards

Medications on the Four Dollar List are often considered new or name brand medications. May even be medications that are seen on television as "ask your provider if it is right for you" medications. These medications can be pricey to the patient.

Patients can

- View the website for discount or coupons for medications

- Check with pharmacies to see if there are any discount cards for medications.

- Ask your provider if they have any discount medication cards that will cover the medication

- Contact the company making the medication and see if they offer any assistance on the medication or any samples.

All ways to get help paying for medications that are expensive.

Patients Get Insurance Books

Welcome to the wonderful world of health insurance. Now here is the insurance book that has all the information you need.

Except that you do not have a clue who to pick for your care out of all the names listed in the book. So what do you do next?

First need is a primary care provider. This is a person who can do all the base care for you. This is the person who will make sure you have base labs, medications for acute and chronic illnesses, regular checkups, annual test, referrals to specialist, and your go to person for health care.

Look in your book and call the provider's offices to see if they are taking new patients. What? Their name is in the book. True, but that does not mean they are accepting new patients. Once a provider accepts insurance, their name will be listed but they may not have any more room for new patients in their schedule.

Once you find a provider that is accepting new patients. Give them a call and set up an appointment.

Next on the list, if you wish to have any specialist, such as for women's care, allergies, and so forth, give those providers a call as well. Then, take this information to your primary care provider. Your primary care provider then can send over a referral.

A referral is basic information from your providers' office such as insurance policy information, identification, and what health problem that needs addressed by the specialist. Example, follow up on allergies that might need more focused care like testing to find out what type of allergies. The specialist will then send your primary care provider any changes they have made in your care to keep everyone in the loop per say.

Your insurance book will be a wealth of information. Books and information typically go out to newly insurance and once a year per insurance company requirements. Many will send out books in the fall. So watch for yours in your mail!

Insurance Deductibles Come First.

What do you mean I owe you? My insurance is supposed to pay that. Right?

Deductibles allow patients to have low insurance payments and still get covered when they need it. Just one catch with those low payments. High deductibles.

Health insurance deductibles work like car insurance deductibles.

Example: The ideas is to pay $100 for car insurance. The insurance company says sure but IF you have an accident, you will have to pay $1000 first before we will fix your car. So you put back $1000 bucks in the bank for when IF happens. IF never happens, no $1000 needed.

Health insurance deductibles are the same thing. Take out the word car and replace it with the word health.

The ideas is to pay $100 for health insurance. The insurance company says sure but IF you have an accident, you will have to pay $1000 first. So you put back $1000 bucks in the bank for when IF happens. IF never happens, no $1000 needed.

Who gets the $1000? This may change per insurance company. With the car it may go to either the insurance company or the mechanic who is going to fix your car.

With the health insurance, it may go to the provider or hospital giving the care or the insurance company may expect the check, giving you instant credit toward your provider's care and insurance paying kicks in to start paying the bills. Patients need to read the fine print to avoid OMG moments later when payments are demanded.

Paying Insurance Co-Payments

Your insurance co-payment (co-pay) is always due at the time of your visit. What does this mean? Your insurance co-payment may be a fixed price or a changing price depending on who you are seeing.

A co-payment is an agreement the patient makes with the insurance company when paying or purchasing insurance.

Example: A co-payment is much like when you go out to dinner with a friend. The check comes and the agreement is to split the bill a certain way. Co-payments are agreements to split the insurance bill. Patients may agree to pay $20 and the insurance company pays the rest to the provider. The insurance company will get the rest of the bill for the patient minus the co-payment amount paid.

No co-payments mean that there is zero amount due and the insurance company is paying for the visit.

But if your provider ask for a co-payment, that amount needs to be paid.

Often, patients will get angry about paying a co-payments. This means that they do not understand what a co-payment agreement is. It is not an agreement with your provider and you, it was set up between your insurance company and you. Once patients realize this, they will pay the co-payment.

Write Off Insurance Paid Bills

Tax time is when all those insurance bills paid may make a difference or not. Depending on the tax code changes, insurance bills may or may not be written off.

The difference is if the establishment providing services is for profit or a nonprofit.

There is one time when insurance bills may qualify for write offs on tax forms. When the care was provided by a nonprofit hospital or medical business. When paying for the service rendered to a nonprofit, keep your documentation stating the bill was paid and then consult your tax advisor.

Depending on your taxes, this can make a difference in taxes due and overpayments resulting in refunds.
This is why many patients will frequent a nonprofit hospital over a for profit hospital.

Nonprofits qualifying for United States Federal write offs will need to be registered with the Internal Revenue Services (IRS). States may also qualify nonprofits but those organizations may not have Federal registration in addition. The laws may very at the states level. It is always wise to check for qualifications.

Ten Percent Donation

It is tax time again! Yuk! Right? I know! But, hey! Couture Health Care can help! Couture Health Care accepts donations in any size! We can help you reach your spiritual and religious tidings of 10% at tax time. Look at your taxes and see if you are giving to meet your spiritual needs or not. If not, contact us and see how we can help you. We are registered with the IRS as a 501c3 nonprofit and the first of our type in the entire United States!

Couture Health Care is just more than a "doctor office". We accept patients for who they are and where they are in life. We accept self pays, flat rates, concierge packages, insurance, and on really hungry days, you might be able to barter services by providing the office lunch. Yeah, we are that cool.

Not just cool, but awesome too. We offer spiritual care for the distressed and those dealing with hard life problems. AND we don't just stop there, if you need health care, we can provide this too.

Dr. Lisa Goins is a licensed Clergy in the State of Ohio, holds an Advance Practice Nurse and Registered Nurse licenses with a board certification in Family Practice as a Nurse Practitioner. And on top of all that she has a doctoral degree in holistic heal and is a Reiki, Master, and Teacher. So now you can get care and meet your spiritual or religious tidings %! Call the office to make an appointment at 513-857-5679 or check out the website at **www.couturehealthcare.org**

Health Care Savings with Health Care Accounts

Health Care Accounts can be a win-win for patients. Health Care Accounts allow individuals to put money in an account that is pre-taxed. This money is then used for health care needs, such as paying for glasses, diabetic supplies, shoes, and general health care needs.

This account can be very beneficial for those looking to save money on their health care expenses.

Health Care Accounts do have restrictions. Individuals may need to purchase and be reimbursed by their accounts. Individuals may need to use a special debit card when purchasing items that are approved.

Health Care Accounts may not roll over from one year to the next. This means that any money saved back will be lost if not spent during the time frame.

Health Care Accounts are good to have if a patient has a chronic illness or part of a large family with many medical needs. The savings of pre-taxed dollars may help families trying to figure out how to stretch their financial needs for health care cost.

Health Care Savings with Health Maintenance

Many individuals do not seek regular health care or visit a provider every year for checkups. Getting a checkup lets the individual know if there are any concerns or changes needed for their health. Yet, many individuals do not frequent a provider and will wait until something major happens.

Once a major event happens, this is when the individual may find out that the incident may have been prevented with routine care or that routine care is now necessary for the rest of the life. This can be very shocking to the individual and may interrupt the course of life, job, and finances.

Routine health care will include yearly blood work, vital signs, may include vitamins, and vaccine updates. A little bit of prevention will help keep your health at excellent levels.

Health Care Savings with Cash.

Many providers will accept cash for payment for a visit. What makes this unique is that if the cash is paid at the time of visit, may be cheaper for the individual, who does not have insurance. Paying at the time of the visit may include any discount rates for cash paid services or bundled services with the visit.

Other services offered may be concierge services or packages. These services may include visits with bundled services to the individuals' home or office. There may be a pre-paid fee per month or year for the retainer of the provider and then another fee when the provider shows up.

Another cash service is a flat fee rate. This is the cost of visit and may or not have bundled services. The rate may be the same as one paid by anyone in the office on a first visit or the equivalent to what would be received by the provider for a visit paid for insurance. Rates can vary per provider.

Health Care Savings with Insurance

Everyone wants to save money and one way to save money is with insurance. Insurance can save you money in a serious event. It can make your health care cost lower or not at all, depending on what type of insurance.

One way to ensure that an individual is getting their worth out of their insurance is to be sure that the type of insurance is accepted by the provider or network of individuals frequented by the individual.

It the health provider does not take the insurance, the individual will be billed for the visit.

So before signing on to an insurance, give your provider a call to see if they accept the insurance. It may save switching to another provider or paying the bill out of pocket. Should an individual be ready to accept their Medicare, this is extremely important, since many choose an insurance their long time provider does not accept. This causes the individual to find a new provider.

Health Care Savings with a Medicine Closet

There are times of the year when things go on sale and can be picked up a low prices. This is a good time to make sure your medicine closet has everything it needs. Check your expirations once a year and do not keep medicines in bathrooms. Moisture will cause medications to weaken by changing their structures. Keeping medications outside the bathroom will also prevent accidental overdose and visitors using your prescription doses without your consent that may not be in their best interest.

Medicine closets may include and not limited to:
Bandages of different sizes
Isopropyl alcohol
Peroxide
Anti-bacterial ointment
Anti-pyretic (fever) and pain medications
Thermometer
Cotton balls
Scissors
Blood pressure cuff
Each medicine closet will have different supplies but all should care a basic first aid kit.

Any assortment of medications, should be labeled, such as; eye, pain, stomach, sinuses, and so forth. This can help when an individual is sick and easily find the medication that will make them feel better. It can also be found by someone with direction in an emergency.

Dyslexia and Test Taking

Dyslexia is difficulty in learning to read due to the problems with interpreting letters, words, numbers, and symbols correctly. Individuals having this problem find that their anxiety increases tenfold.

The difficult in learning new material may be an increasing challenge but then a major life changing test or exam can bring on a panic attack in an individual with dyslexia.

Increased stress and anxiety can over load and over stimulate the individual with dyslexia and decrease functional output of quality work and results on test and exams. External room stimuli, others in the room with limited noise, and the inability to focus on words on paper or computer to get the meaning will inadvertently cause the individual to fail the exam.

Tips that made help.

- Request individual rooms for test taking.

- Wear ear plugs and sounds silencing head gear.

- Take a few minutes to familiarize yourself with the test. Read over the entire paper test or do the computer tutorial. It will give time to become comfortable and relax some before the starting the actual test or exam.

- Request extra time or no time limit for the exam. This will help decrease some anxiety related to a timed test.

- Limit all caffeine the week of the major exam if not wean off completely. This will help prevent faulty increasing anxiety.

- Eat well before all test and exams. Long test demand brain power. Cells need fuel for hours and hours of testing. Fruits break down into simple sugars and will be used quickly. Protein and carbohydrates take longer to break down.

- Read the statement, information, and questions to the punctuation marks. Re-read three times to make sure that

- you comprehend the exam question. Not reading the question correctly buy ignoring the pause by a comma can cause incorrect answers to be chosen.

- Understand that the answer is in front of you on multiply choice questions.

- Do not over think or add to the question. Your own experiences may not apply to the question and you will select an answer that should be right but not the answer to the question. The computer only cares what the answer it is told is right by the programmer. It will not argue your ideas.

- Reverse the test/exam. Review the answers first and then read the question.

- Sleep as much as you can the week before the test. This will prevent exhaustion if you just cannot sleep the night before the test/exam.

- Drink plenty of water the week of the exam. Hydration of brain cells keeps the brain alert.

- Limit outside stresses or enhancing unnecessary stress. Hold off on external stresses if possible. Before major exams, adults may want to "get their house in order" meaning all bills paid and household cleaning done to keep stress down. Children may need to limit television, gaming, extra events, excessive toys, and stressful family events before major testing. Children may also need to eat more on days of testing to ensure enough brain power for desired results.

Dyslexia and Sleep

Dyslexia is difficulty in learning to read due to the problems with interpreting letters, words, numbers, and symbols correctly. The question then becomes, what can make it worse? Lack of quality sleep for a person with dyslexia can make everything affected by dyslexia worse. A lot worse. Everything becomes harder. In young children this can cause behavior problems. Melt downs, crying, withdrawing from task, and grades will suffer.

Those adults with dyslexia will find that a poor night's sleep will result in poor performance at work. Adults will try to compensate with beverages to increase their functioning abilities but they will be more alert and able to verbally function but may lack core resources to produce quality texted work. Adults will come back days later and review a task, only to notice the poor quality and be of concern, if not pointed out by another earlier on.

In the lack of sleep phase, dyslexic twisting of fonts and numbers that will seem perfectly right to the dyslexic when in a well-rested phase, the work and quality will be different.
Thus, to improve and limit difficulty with dyslexia, increase rest and sleep will not make the disability go away but it will lessen the affect it has on the individual.

Dyslexia and Colors

Dyslexia is difficulty in learning to read due to the problems with interpreting letters, words, numbers, and symbols correctly. This does not mean that the person with dyslexia has a problem with intelligence.

It does mean that the learning curve to gain knowledge is hampered by the inability to increase intelligence by reading for knowledge. It is not uncommon for a person with dyslexia to read a paragraph and not retain what they read due to the difficulty of trying to figure out what each word or string of words says.

Here is a study tip that may help someone with dyslexia.

- Color the words to help trigger remembering.

Example: Systems of the body can be colorized. Blood is red. Respiratory is blue. Urinary system is yellow. When recalling the words, colors will help trigger the right response.

Dyslexia and Chunking

What is dyslexia? Dyslexia is difficulty in learning to read due to the problems with interpreting letters, words, numbers, and symbols correctly. This does not mean that the person with dyslexia has a problem with intelligence.

One of the problems with remembering a lot of material or a sequence of events, is a problem for a dyslexic person. One way to do this is chunking. What is chunking? Chunking is when you take lots of material and only focus on the first part to remember it, then move to the second part, and so forth. Example of chunking is social security numbers and telephone numbers 000-00-0000 and 555-555-5555.

Chunking is a way to learning for a dyslexic person.

Example:
Let us exam the standard page with three paragraphs on it.

- There is a beginning, middle, and ending paragraph.

- Ready the first paragraph and stop.

- What were the key words? Avoid the filler or fluff words such as; A, the, and, so forth. What are the nouns or subjects and then the verbs or action words? This will help with comprehension.

- Repeat with the second paragraph.

- What content does it add to the topic? Or does it start a new topic?

- Is there more information added to the content from the first paragraph?

- Repeat with the third paragraph.

- Adding the main content to the first and second paragraphs, there should be a completed thought, story, and idea with a conclusion.

Studying Example:
Studying is an evasive idea to someone who has dyslexia. How does one study. Often, many students do not understand how to or what it means to study. Study is not memorizing but learning a concept, idea, or material to retain not just for the test but for recall in a career.

Chunking used to study.

- Start at the first paragraph. Focus on the key words, nouns, verbs, and concept.

- Do this for only twenty minutes. Take a break. Test yourself on what you know by verbalizing it to another or writing out what you remember.

- Begin again, but this time start at the end of the last paragraph and move to the second paragraph. This will help tie in paragraph one and two ideas, thoughts, and information. Then stop after twenty minutes.

- Repeat with paragraph three.

By chunking the information and giving breaks to test the retaining of information, will help a dyslexic to remember a lot of valuable information for the long term.

Dyslexia and Your Other Left

How many times have you been told, it is your other left? If you had one dollar for everyone who has said this to you, that you would be well beyond rich. Why is this? What is dyslexia?

Dyslexia is difficulty in learning to read due to the problems with interpreting letters, words, numbers, and symbols correctly.

This does not mean that the person with dyslexia has a problem with intelligence. In does mean that learning may take longer than a person without dyslexia. The learning curve may be overwhelming to them at first. It will take longer for them to read, understand, and digest the material for recall.

So this brings in the other left. There is a simple way to test for dyslexia and it is called the clock test. It deals with numbers and spacing. Most everyone has seen a clock face and understands that the numbers go around in a circle from one to twelve. Everyone knows there is spacing to make this happen. The test involves the individual to write the numbers down in order around the circle. Very simple test.

The outcomes for positive results for dyslexia will show that the numbers nine to twelve will be squished together or even omitting numbers of ten or eleven to make it all fit. Why is this? The brain will block out the left side and visual area. Those with dyslexia will often ignore their upper left side of vision.

Takes training to remember "your other left" because the right is dominate in society but the dyslexic may be naturally left but has been trained that right is acceptable. So when told left, the dyslexic person will have to pause and think what is the difference between right and left. Thus, selecting the correct left.

This may be why reading in some languages becomes a problem. Reading will start from left to right. Thus, focusing in a difficult area and then trying to retain information from it.

One solution is to take reading material and move it more to the clock patter of one to six area or turning the book at an angle to read. This helps keep the material in a focused region of interest and makes the learning easier.

Quitting Smoking with a New Habit

Smoking is a habit. It took time to practice lighting up, inhaling the smoke, flicking the ashes, and putting out the cigarette. The individual had to learn where to pick up a pack of cigarettes or purchase a box to make smoking cigarettes easier to access.

After time, smoking cigarettes became something the individual did and it was now a current life style choice. At this point, the effects of smoking may have gone un-noticed by the smoker after many years of just lighting up. Smokers may even seek out others, who also smoke. Activities will be started or joined just so smoking may happen.

Until the day the individual decides to stop smoking. Then this habit becomes one that needs to be broken.

Undoing a habit of putting the hand to the mouth with a cigarette will need to be replaced with another habit. Many make a choice of using food and regret this choice twenty pounds later.

Picking a healthy habit may be daunting but there is one that is cheap, available, and the hand to mouth isn't a problem. That habit is drinking water.

Water helps flush the system and freshens the body. Drinking water instead of smoking will help decrease the nicotine in the body. Making it even easier to quit smoking. Water will help clear the mind, hydrate the body and skin, and decrease the need to over eat.

Quitting Smoking with Medications

Quitting smoking is always on the mind of someone who smokes. When the time comes for the smoker to commit to quit smoking, is when the smoker will be the most successful. The smoker has to want to stop smoking.

Now that does not make it easy to quit smoking. There is much research to show that smoking is addicting due to the chemicals in cigarettes. This addiction is what gives the difficulties in going cold turkey or putting the cigarettes down and never lighting up.

Many smokers turn to medications. There are many times and each medication used may have side effects. The trouble with selecting medications is not the form of choice, such as, chewing gum, patches, or fake cigarettes. It is matching the medication to the smoker. Many medications are equal to a number of cigarettes smoked. Too much or too little medication can ruin a sincere attempt at quitting. Other problems that can arise is complications with other medications taken by the smoker.

It is always a good idea to check with your provider on avoiding products that can interfere with current medications and avoiding adverse side effects.

Quitting Smoking with Others

Quitting Smoking is called cessation of smoking. A lot of smokers like to smoke with each other. Many smokers will light up at their breaks. Many will smoke two cigarettes each break. Two breaks during an eight hour day is four cigarettes. Four cigarettes times five days of work is twenty cigarettes. Typically in a regular pack of cigarettes is twenty cigarettes. One pack of cigarettes smoked just at breaks at work.

So during a fifteen minute break at work, each cigarette is about 5-7 minutes in time to smoke. So what happens when you hold that first cigarette 5-7 minutes long and not smoke it? You just cut out ten cigarettes out per week. Half a pack of smokes.

So hold that cigarette, do some talking or wait until the co-worker lights up cigarette number two on break. Then light up. Again, only half a pack of smokes cut out.

As this becomes more comfortable, cut out the smoking completely on one of the breaks. The follow it by not smoking at any breaks. Suddenly, you are down on pack of smokes a week.

Quitting Smoking by Removing One

Quitting smoking is called cessation of smoking. It is not an easy task to do when one has been smoking most of their life. But there are things you can do to slow down or easy up on the habit.

Here is the tip to help you begin cutting back as you smoke.
In a regular packet of cigarettes, there are twenty cigarettes.

When you open the pack, remove one cigarette. Now if you smoke a pack a week, this is one cigarette a week. If you smoke a pack a day, then it is seven cigarettes a week you have just stopped smoking. Pretty awesome right?

Now let us do the math. One cigarette equals one week. Twenty cigarettes equals twenty weeks or four months. Thus, on week two, you remove two cigarettes from the pack. Week three, you will remove three cigarettes per pack and keep doing this until you get down to week twenty.

At this point it is going to be easy to lay the pack down.

Quit Smoking by Smoking

Quitting smoking is called cessation of smoking. There are many ways to quit but some involve time, money, effort, and many just can't do it.

Did you know you can stop smoking by just smoking? The trick is that you can't do anything else. When you light up to smoke. You can't do any other task but smoke.

A lot of smokers bought into the advertisement to smoke while doing activities. It was to make them look cool. What it really did was hide the fact that many folks will increase smoking or letting their smokes burn up in an ashtray. Marketing win to buy more smokes and make the company money.

So just smoke. Do not do anything else. What people notice happens when they do this, they do not smoke nearly as many cigarettes during the day.

Just focusing on doing nothing but smoking will actually help cut down on smoking.

Prepare to be an Ex-Smoker

Three ways to prepare to become an ex-smoker.

Brush teeth and/or use mouth wash after smoking. This will help decrease the taste of smoke in the mouth.

Wear freshly washed clothes and prevent wearing clothes that smell like smoke. This will help train the mind into finding the smell distasteful.

Clean all the carpets, furniture, and drapes in your home. The fresh smell and lack of smoke will be noticeable. If you smoke outside, make sure you are doing it far from your doors. Let your laziness work for you. If it becomes too much effort to get dressed to go outside to smoke, you will not smoke.

Smoke Less in a Month

Remove one cigarette every week from your cigarette pack. Continue until you have no cigarettes in your pack left to smoke.

Based on a one pack a week habit, this will take 20 weeks to stop smoking. At a one pack a day, remove the same number of cigarettes from the pack for the week.

On average a pack of cigarettes hold 20 individual cigarettes. If you smoke a pack a day, then removing one cigarette from the pack and not smoking it, will have decreased you smoking by 1 cigarette daily, 7 for the week, and 30 for the month. A pack and a half less smoking over the month.

Then, by increasing the following week by taking 2 out the packet, the results double.

Three Ways to Quit Smoking

Hold the cigarette and do not light it. This will slow down your smoking and may limit smoking by one cigarette. Many times the first cigarette lit up will be quickly smoked and another one lit up before the person realizes they are on the second cigarette. Just slowing down can limit cigarettes smoked.

Focus on smoking. Do not do any other activities other than smoking. This prevents smoking more than necessary. Many times when someone lights up a cigarette they are busy multi-tasking and not even realizing they are smoking several cigarettes. By focusing on smoking and not multi-tasking, the amount of cigarettes will decrease.

Begin to find other ways to replace smoking before you light up. Take a walk, do arm exercises, and so forth. You are replacing the habit with another. Eventually, you will limit the cigarettes you light up because you have replaced the habit of smoking with the habit of walking or other exercises.

Depression and Vitamin D3

Depression symptoms may need intervention with medications. Often there are times when prescription medications may not be possible for the individual to take.

Another option for depression is Vitamin D3. Vitamin D3 levels should be checked by a provider. This will help determine the dose of Vitamin D3.

Vitamin D3 helps with depression and anxiety. Vitamin D3 is a fat soluble vitamin and this means it takes time to build up in the human body. If levels are below normal, it will take several weeks to reach normal levels. This means that if the level is low, the Vitamin D3 will need to be a correcting dose. This is to get the Vitamin D3 to normal. If the Vitamin D3 level is normal, then a maintenance does is needed.

Vitamin D3 should be taken at breakfast or by lunch due to the long half-life. If taken too late in the day, may cause insomnia. If the individual works nights, then Vitamin D3 needs to be taken before leaving for work.

Many insurances will cover the cost of Vitamin D3. Vitamin D3 is available for purchase over the counter in different doses.

Depression Risk for Suicide

Depression's hopelessness and despair can lead one to believe that suicide is the answer to escape their misery, pain, and make it go away.

Warning signs include; talking about harming or killing self, taking about their death and dying, reckless behavior, saying goodbye and getting affairs in order, statements in the past tense, and mood changes.

Individuals with plans for suicide may have the means or not. Intervention is needed for the individual. The individual may need to go to the Emergency room and let them know they do not feel safe and why. They may be admitted for observation and intervention.

Providers may be contacted and may help streamline interventions with mental health agencies for therapy and treatment.

Depression Signs and Symptoms

What is depression? What are the signs and symptoms of depression?

Those who feel depressed may feel hopeless and helpless to do things. They feel things will not get better and they have no control over changing their situation. This will result in a loss of activities and participation in things that use to bring them joy. The lack of involvement in activities may lead to overeating or eating less. This will result in a sudden weight gain or loss in weight. They may miss meals or not care if it is meal time.

Changes in going to bed to sleep, getting up, napping during the day. Some may find they wake too early or over sleep. The changes in sleep may cause irritability and tolerance in others. The lack of sleep may lead to feeling fatigue, exhausted, or just drained of energy. Everyday chores and tasks take forever to complete.

Concentration becomes a problem in completing tasks and remembering things. Recklessness may happen leading to preventable accidents. Non-accident problems may include headaches, joint and pains, including stomach trouble.
If you are experiencing signs and symptoms of depression, contact your provider to discuss your symptoms.

Depression

Depression is a form of sadness that may last for several weeks to several months.

How do I know if I have depression?

Providers ask patients several questions to help determine if patients are depressed.

- Do you feel hopeless or helpless?

- Have you lost interest in things you enjoy? This includes being with friends and involvement in activities.

This short screening of questions can help the provider determine if you are depressed. Patients that say yes to these questions may be suffering from depression.
The provider may continue with more questions to discern more information about the depression and target in on a treatment that will benefit the patient best.

- Do you feel rested or are you tired all the time?

- Has your sleeping and eating habits changed?

- Do you find you have trouble with easy task? Concentration is harder now?

- You are not positive and you cannot shake your negative thoughts?

- Behavior has become irritable, aggressive, and you get mad easy?

- Behavior includes recklessness activities and increase in alcohol.

The rest of the questions will help the provider to decide on what therapy and treatments may work best for you.
If you find yourself saying yes to these questions please call your provider. Often times, depression may have resulted from a life changing event, may be a result from current medications, or another underlying medical problem undiagnosed.

First Responders Preparations

First responders are those who are on the seen first. First responders may have seen the event unfold or not. They may or not always know how to care for the event unfolding.
What can you do to prepare?

- Learn to access your 911 quickly in your areas and show others. Learn what to say, such as, explaining the area you are in, what is going on, and other valuable information that will help the 911 operator send correct help.

- Learn CPR. There may be those who are in need after an event has happen.

- Learn how to be safe. Avoid power lines, water outlets, shooters, and other events.

- Learn basic first aid.

- Learn how to find emergency equipment. AEDS, Fire Extinguishers, and Safe locations.

- Understand that first responders may also be in danger.

Avoid being a problem, be the solution. If you cannot help, step back and let someone else.

First Responders Emotions

First responders are those who are on the seen first. First responders may have seen the event unfold or not. They may or not always know how to care for the event unfolding.

- Emotions will vary as adrenaline is in effect.

- Try to remain calm and think.

- Call 911 and give information. Do not hang up, if you cannot safely talk. Do not assume someone else will.

- Move to safety.

- Take others with you to safety, if possible.

- Remove any barriers to safety if necessary.

- Slow and stop all bleeding. Give CPR.

Individuals may respond differently than you. There is no wrong or right.
If you are of no help or cannot help, step aside and let someone else do it.

First Responders to Public Shooting Events

First responders are those who are on the seen first. First responders may have seen the event unfold or not. They may or not always know how to care for the event unfolding.

1. Call 911. Give information if possible. Do not hang up. 911 can track the call and send help.

2. Move to safety. If possible, take as many with you as possible.

3. Do not go back into the area of danger for anything.

4. Care for yourself first. Be the solution, not the problem.

5. Care for others.

6. Give CPR if necessary or slow/stop bleeding of those around you.

7. Step back and let help take over when they arrive.

Provide information to emergency help when asked. Tell them what happen and what you have done to help any individuals.

First Responder for Shot Gun Wounds

First responders are those who are on the seen first. First responders may have seen the event unfold or not. They may or not always know how to care for the event unfolding.

1. Ensure safety. Move to safety if possible.

2. Stay calm. Calmness allows to thinking and care to be given.

3. Call 911 or for help.

4. Check for a pulse, if the person is not actively moving or talking.

5. Check for terminal wounds. These are wounds that need immediate attention. Head and chest wounds.

6. Cover wounds with hands or fabric/cloth. Applying pressure to wounds will slow/stop the bleeding.

7. Keep the individual alert and talking.

8. When help arrives, step back, and let them take over.

First responders may need to give any information to those who arrive from the 911 call. This may include any contact information from the responder.

Summer Time Shut In

There are times when you just cannot get out in the sun. The reasons can be many from reactions to light sensitive medications to pesky bugs. Do not let it stop you from enjoying the sun!

- Open up the blinds and curtains. Let the sunshine come to you!

- Sit in patio areas when possible to absorb the sunshine.

- Move office desk near window areas. It will make working inside less miserable on beautiful days.

- Sit and look out the window for a while. It will trick the mind to thinking you did not miss anything.

Summer Time Bone Health

Summer time is a great time to improve bone health. One of the easiest methods is walking.

- Place foot heel first when walking. Avoid placing toes first with stepping down.

- Walk 60 minutes a day.

- Try to walk outside when possible.

- Wear supportive shoes to prevent injuries.

- Take a friend when possible. Buddy systems strengthen routines and makes it fun.

Several months of summer time walking will help build up bone health for fall and winter.

Summer Time FREE Vitamin D

Summer is a great time to get lots of Vitamin D. Increased levels of Vitamin D can improve mood, bone strength, decrease anxiety and depression, and much more.

Where can you get FREE Vitamin D? Just step out in the sun! Yes. Your awesome human body can take the sunshine and convert it into Vitamin D for your body. This is the reason sunbathers enjoy the sun so much. It feels good to their bones.

Side effect of FREE Vitamin D? Sunburn. Application of sunscreen will keep the human body from burning but it will also prevent absorption of Vitamin D. Other ways to avoid sunburn is step out in the sun in the early hours or later hours for fifteen minutes a day.

Want Fabulous Hair?

Look at your vitamin B intake. Vitamin B is a water soluble vitamin. This means it needs to be replenished in the diet or with supplement vitamins. It is always better to get your vitamins via your intake of food and calories.

Sometimes, the food that is eaten is not always packed with vitamins or minerals. In this case, a supplement may be necessary.

Vitamin B can help with hair and nail growth, increase energy levels, and improve overall mood.

Vitamin B levels can be tested. The most common test are for Vitamin B12 and Vitamin B6.

It may take several weeks to notice the results and in several months new hair and nails will be noticeable.

Summer Time Vitamins

Summer is a great time to improve your health. One way to start is to increase your immunity health.

Vitamins are divided into water and fat soluble types.

- A vitamin that is considered water soluble is one that needs to be replenished daily. Vitamin C is a water soluble vitamin.

- A vitamin that is a fat soluble is one that that builds up in the body over time. Vitamin D 3 is a fat soluble vitamin

A multi vitamin is a combination of all vitamins and include minerals. This version will consist of a selection of vitamins based on their daily allowance.

Individual vitamins or supplements may come in increased amounts. These types are used to maintain a vitamin level in the body or increase the amount of vitamin level in the body to correct a low amount in the body.

Vitamins take time to build up in the body. This is why starting vitamins in the summer is great. Several months of vitamins can build up immunity and help stop or keep illnesses away in the fall and winter months.

Annual Mother's Day Pass It Forward

Mother's Day is an annual first Sunday in May. Surprise, it also happens the same time flowers can be planted. Appliances go on sale, what Mom don't need another kitchen gadget? Not to mention the jewelry and food coupons that saturate the market. Mother's Day is the biggest day outside Christmas that dumps lots of cash in the market. Maybe this is why the stock markets begin selling off in May? Just how much are you spending on Mom? Not enough, if you talk to advertisers.

Even sadder is those Moms that have passed away. Kids still feel the need to purchase stuff and place it on their graves. While wonderful and meaningful…it really is not. It is hard to mow over Mom's grave so the graveyard attendants pick up the stuff and toss it in the trash. Sometimes the dumpster divers get it and re-sell it or the bolder ones just take it off the graves after you leave.

So instead of the mandatory trip to the store to buy Mom something that she may not really need or use, instead do something awesome.

This year, pass it forward. Do something awesome for someone in honor of Mom. Show others how well you were raised. But if you do have to "spend" on Mom, "spend" some time with her.

Forever Christmas

I have worked in many a nursing home over my many years in nursing. One thing I have noticed and many others have as well, is the forever Christmas season. Why is this?

Many residents are elderly. What does elderly mean? There are two spans of elderly. The age from 65-85 and 85 and up. To realize what this means, if a resident is 85 and up, their children may be 20 years their junior or younger. Their children are also considered elderly. If a lady is 100, her adult child may be 80. This may be the reason that staff will not see family coming in. Often, staff will see grandchildren and great-grandchildren, elders of the church, and very long time friends that will visit.

This also means that often the time of visiting may not be regular but during seasonal events, such as Christmas. What do you get someone in a nursing home? Christmas stuff. Things like a Christmas tree, socks, clothes, and holiday blankets. Many times, these belongs will be the only belongs a resident of a nursing home has and they will not want to put them away just because Christmas is over. They will say, so-and-so gave that to me. Leave it up or I will wear that today.

Now you know why there is forever Christmas.

Breakfast is Important

Breakfast. Why is it so important? Let us explore the word a bit. Breakfast use to be two words, not one word. It was break fast. Fast was what you did when you did not eat for a long period of time. To breaking fast, you ate a meal of particular foods to energize you until your next meal.

The next meal normally was around noon. Noon was when the sun was high overhead and often too hot to work outside. People would stop around noon to drink fluids and eat a meal, waiting for it to cool off outside to continue working. Then the last meal of the day was in the evening hours.

Many of the breaking fast times centered around times when people did chores outside. Getting up to milk the cows, feed the chickens, and take the cattle into the field. Then advertisement got a hold of the words and decided to merge them into one word. Easy to print on products, get the word out there, and eventually accepted to everyone as one word.

So the first meal of the day is breakfast. It does not matter if it is 4 a.m. or 11 a.m. For people that work all night it might be at 5 p.m.

Therefore, the first meal of the day needs to be packed with nutrients, vitamins, fluids, proteins, and carbohydrates. Natural and artificial sugars will break down quickly and get you going. Proteins will then break down, followed by carbohydrates into the body.

The balance of meals with too many carbohydrates will keep the body's fuel stagnate and will end up building up in the system. This causes weight gain in a body that is not as active as it needs to be. Too many sugars and the body has lots of energy but then burns out. People who say, they do not eat breakfast, really are saying they do not eat in the morning hours. They do eat breaking fast meals.

500 Calorie Give Away Diet Plan

Many people do not even know where to begin when losing weight. They can see and are fully aware they are overweight. No need from society for the constant reminder. What is needed is help, support, and ideas.
500 Calories is where to start.

On average, 250 calories is needed to be eliminated from the diet daily to lose weight. Now a diet is what you eat every day. Diet is now used by marketing to imply weight loss or what type of food consumption, such as Paleo diet, Diabetic diet, and Vegan diet.

Removing 250 calories is equal to a standard size chocolate bar. So removing 500 calories does not seem to be that much, correct?
500 Calorie Give Away Diet is easy.
500 calories x 7 days is 2,100 calories removed a week. This should result in one to two pounds lost.
So how can you remove 500 calories a day?

- Two chocolate bars

- Two cans of regular soda/pop

- Sides, such as fries.

- Downsize meal to regular size.

- No extras or condiments

- No seconds, thirds, or entire box.

- Small cups, plates or bowls, pots/pans, spoons, etc.

- Stop when you are full and put the food away.

- Stop eating and doing other things.

- Eat half of what is ordered for fast food.

Many ways to remove 500 calories and no need to weight to tomorrow to start.

Disclaimer: The bigger BMI (30 and up) will see better results and find this effective for the individual. Individuals in their BMI range, who need to take off a few pounds, will not see a lot of success because they are already within the calorie ranges for their body types.

Weight Loss By Counting Calories

Weight loss can be done by counting calories. That said, there are factors that need to be adjusted to prevent failure from happening with weight loss.

- Realistic expectations of how many calories that are already consumed daily.

- Types of foods eaten to get the calories already consumed daily.

- Refusal of trying new foods.

- Inability to eat foods, such as allergies or intolerance to a type of food.

- The total of calories that make up non-food items consumed, such as beverages from beer to soda/pop.

- Access to food types. Budgets do not let everyone eat nutritious meals frequently.

- Additives to foods can count for many calories.

On average, removing 250 calories daily from consuming can result in one pound a week lost. Those who cut more calories will see more weight loss.

Average calories are 1,800 to 2,000 total per day consumed for 12,600 to 14,000 calories per week.

What makes weight loss so hard is finding out that one meal equals 2,000 calories and expecting two more meals that day. It can be quite a struggle to lose weight and give up.

What can work? Removing calories from each meal daily. Decide on how many calories to forgo each meal. For math sake, let us say 100 calories each meal. That will be more than 250 per day. To give you an idea on the 250 calories, that is a standard chocolate bar. If you eat one a day and then stop, weight loss would be one pound a week. One eight ounce regular soda/pop is 100-180 calories. See how easy it would be to not just each that one more thing?

Remove from each meal

- Do not order supersize/big drinks. Order small. Many smalls were the 1970's larges. They hold 8 to 16 ounces. That is one to two servings.

- No sides. Sides can be several hundred calories.

- Watch the dressings and extras. Check out the calorie count. You will be surprised.

- Condiments. Hidden calories here up to 70 calories or more if not careful.

- Remove one slice of bread. That is 140 to 70 calories.

- Eat half the serving. Often the serving order is three or four servings.

- Downsize the entire meal. Eat on smaller plates or in bowls.

- Downsize the cups, serving spoons, and cooking pots. Your eyes will want to fill up a pot but your pot is now not as big.

Counting calories this way does not change the way you eat completely but it gives you a start you can see on the scales.

Boots and Siblings

When the military adult child or significant other comes home for a visit after being gone a long time, there is a rush to meet up with everyone. Younger adult military visiting home may have siblings at home that may not understand the importance of the time and visit. Time is moments and time is short. Siblings may get jealous of the preferences and the lack of attention from parents. Parents need to set aside time for the siblings or explain the special significance of the visit.

Older siblings may be traveling in to visit or meet up. Again, there may be jealous or resentment as the military person gets more attention, especially if they have also traveled and been away a long time as well. Parents will need to divide attention and set up time to be with each child and together. Eating a meal together verses spending time with each one doing adult events may meet everyone's needs.

Parents may experience a lot of emotions. This is normal. It may have been awhile since the house was full and they had gotten use to the quite, which is now destroyed. Parents also need to keep up with their routine of sleeping, exercising, and eating meals, all while realizing that the upsetting of their homeostasis is temporary.

Boots and Boxes

Many families of military adult children and significant others, often feel that life is full of boxes.

During a military career, it seems that everyone knows the shipping price of a box and gets really good at Tetris by packing everything into a space with six folds. For many significant others and parents, this is the first time to get the "kid in a box" home. Some parents find it interesting to see what their adult child has sent home.

Sometimes there might be a note scribbled on the box. The box may be full of everything they brought with them to start their career and then finding they do not need it to just getting an envelope with some information. Often in this case, it is that the adult child has donated everything to a good cause and decided it would be better used if donated than sent home.

Later on, the boxes from home begin. Care packages will start. Things from home that can be eaten will be sent. Items that remind the adult child of home will be sent. Even missed holiday goodies will go out many months before the date, to arrive in those hard to reach locations close to holiday time for those serving in the military. Parents and significant others will learn about the lists of dos and don'ts, if not from researching, certainly from trial and errors.

The pro of boxes, is new traditions begin. Messages on the inside of the box will start. Small holiday item traditions will start as the new way things are done because of time and limited space. Things suddenly become more important than ribbons and bows but the content trumps in importance.

Boots In House

Anxious parents cannot wait until their military adult child returns home. Often, the time home is not what the parents expect. Many adult children return home with agendas. Things they want to get done while they are home. The may want to pack up things for deployment, visit friends, hang out with siblings, and sometimes it feels like, the last thing they want to do is hang out with Mom and Dad.

Many military parents have the famous pictures of the sleeping adult child on the couch at their house. The reason why an adult child may have traveled several time zones or half way around the world to see them. Jet lag is a problem that can cut into a visit home.

Over scheduling is another huge problem. Parents and the adult child both tend to over schedule plans and then get frustrated when plans change. Pick out one or two things that both parties agree on, such as, going out to eat and celebrate homecoming or an open house for all family and friends one day during the visit.

Working parents may find that they are not as needed for the time scheduled off, may want to plan a few back up plans for themselves. Things they wanted to get done while off too. This way if the couch has no vacancy, they can make themselves busy with other plans. It is all good.

Baby Shower Vaccines

Awe! A new baby in the family! Congratulations! The new mom-to-be most likely has been updated on her vaccines, as she will be passing on immunity to the baby in the first months of life, but what about the rest of the family? Grandparents-to-be, along with new aunts and uncles, should be sure they are also up to date on their vaccines.

The baby shower is a great time to get everyone on board in getting their vaccine boosters. It gives everyone a chance to get the shot and build immunity before the new baby arrives. Check the 2016 Adult Vaccine list from the Centers of Disease Control (CDC) to see if you are in need of a booster.

http://www.cdc.gov/vaccines/schedules/downloads/adult/adult-combined-schedule.pdf

Adult Child Goes Against Parent's Decision

There is a lot of research on vaccines. As a result of vaccines, there has been a lot of disease go into the history books. This is often why many current generations are concern that their children may or may not get vaccines. Are they necessary? Do they need them? Should they get them? What about a waiver to prevent the need of them?

Here is another concern. Your child's life post 18 years old. Yep, that age when children get the right to do whatever they want and parents cannot stop them. They can smoke, drink, have sex with whoever and whenever, and get vaccinations. Yes, they can reverse some of what you tried to stop them from having. Adult children can change their health history.

Why! Why would they? Because the lack of economic opportunities. The ability to go places and do things may require a needle stick and vaccination to allow them to do it. A good example is being a nurse. Many hospitals mandate a flu vaccine is mandatory and there are no expectations if you want to be employed.

True, a lot of children have been protected by "herd immunity", where everyone else has gotten the vaccine and this protects those who cannot get the vaccine. Yet, more and more are deciding let "herd immunity" handle it. What is happening is outbreaks due to weakness in the "herd immunity".

So while the parent may say no to the vaccinations, the adult child may say yes at 18. Concerned adult children can request a catch up schedule with their providers or the local health department and no, the adult child won't get all of them on the same day. Just like getting the entire series over years, it will take a while to get caught up but not impossible.

Rehome the Family Pets

Sadly there may come a time when the family pet has to be rehomed through no fault of anyone. Rehoming may come about with changes in family, residence, and prevention of neglect of the animal.

How do you find a new forever home for the rehome animal? Getting the word out is to those looking for an older pet. Many forever homes are looking for an animal already trained to use the bathroom box or go outside.

Some forever homes are looking for animals that can stand 24/7 attention from their new loved ones. Many forever homes are looking for animals to take care of because they need a void to fill from the loss of their own animal of many years. Forever homes are already use to having an older animal and welcome the thoughts of taking in an adult animal over a baby animal with care needs that might be just a bit too much for them.

When rehoming the pet, do include any shot records, information on chips, and vet information to the new forever home location. Should an injury to the pet or human be involved, shot records could prevent the pet from getting euthanatized unnecessarily.

Three Reasons Life Is Getting On Your Nerves!

"Dr. Lisa everything is getting on my nerves!" This is a statement that often women will tell me. So let us explore this statement and what I can do.

1. Nerves often are referred to along with anxiety. But is it real anxiety? How much caffeine are we drinking? This is often surprising to a lot of women and men. When they realize that the caffeine overload is what is causing their anxiety.

2. What about food? Do we have heartburn, reflux, GI trouble, and what is diet like? Many times GERD has been confused for anxiety. Why? Because the area of trouble is often in the area of the chest where anxiety can be felt. Many are surprised when GERD medication takes away what they thought was anxiety.

3. One step more, ruling out GERD and anxiety, has there been headaches and what does the blood pressure been? Any jaw, neck, shoulder, back, chest, and arm pain? In the same area of the chest, is the heart. It just might be that the anxiety or nerves is really the heart crying for attention. Often, women ignore this possible diagnosis because they are too young, women, or no real history of problems. A blood pressure medication may solve the solutions.

    Please see a provider when things are getting on your nerves. Depending on where the nerves are talking, it may be a serious problem that needs addressed.

Six Ways To Get Medication Cheaper

"Dr. Lisa, I can't afford my medication! It is just too much!" I have patients tell me this a lot. Paying for medication is a huge concern outside paying for the visit to see a provider. There are some things I can do to help you out.

1. Depending on the medication, I may have samples I can offer. The drawback to the samples have several problems. If the medication is new on the market there may be coupons, discount cards, or offers via the company to get it cheaper. Those items will eventually run out after time and the cost may be way too high without those things keeping it cheap.

2. Switching to generic. This is an instant price cut and often the medication has no changes or effects on the user expect there might be more money in your wallet.

3. Get a prescription for 90 days instead of 30 days. Many pharmacies offer cheaper rates for medications this way. The downside is storing the medication, which can be a problem in a home with varying temperatures and children.

4. The $4 dollar list or whatever the pharmacy wants to call it. This list offers hundreds of medications for 30 days for only $4 dollars. Just ask if your medication is on the $4 dollar list. If it is you can get this price.

5. Switching the medication from a pricy medication to one on the $4 dollar list can save money.

6. Then there are companies/pharmacies that offer FREE medications that can be picked up with a prescription. A limited list but let the provider know and perhaps they can make this happen.

    There are ways to get your medications cheap. Do not let paying for medication put you in the hospital later. A few dollars now can keep the hospital bills away.

Should I keep taking diabetic medication?

"Dr. Lisa, should I keep taking my diabetic medication?" I get asked this question a lot. There are a couple ways we can answer this question.

1. We can take a lab test that is called a hemoglobin A1c. It is a test that tells a story about your cells for the last 120 days. It can be done every 3 to 6 months. The standard guidelines state every six months but every three months can keep better control and better health.

2. Has the individual been implementing any weight loss, exercising, and dietary changes? Yes, it is possible to get off diabetic medication but not always. Some are able to drop lots of weight and retest hemoglobin A1cs and find they no longer qualify them for medication.

3. The other side of this coin is that despite all this work and discipline to control the diabetic number, the hemoglobin A1c number creeps upward anyway. In this case, per standard guidelines current medication may be maxed out, another medication added, and/or insulin needs to be introduced to keep the numbers low.

   Do note that the cells only live 120 days and their story telling does come to an end. If the individual has been working hard on controlling their blood sugars, the results will show up on the next 120 day test.

Fast Pumping, Go!

The most important thing about CPR is doing it. Many folks are afraid to do it and get it wrong. The Good Samaritan law protects anyone from trying to rescue another from law suits.

If you find someone down, unresponsive, and no heart beat is detected, call 911 or point to someone and tell them to call 911.

Then put your hands over each other and over the person's heart. Fast and steady pump down and up on the chest of the unresponsive person. What you are doing is making a heart that has stop, move. This keeps the heart, a pump, pumping blood through the veins.

When 911 support arrives, they will take over. Be proud of yourself! You just became someone's hero!

Three Fast Facts!

Did you know that "normal" blood pressure is under 140/90 and if you are diabetic that "normal" is 130/80?

Did you know that there are four chambers of your heart? Each chamber has a value or "door" to let blood in and out of the chamber. When the "door" does not close it causes the blood to not exit or enter the heart chamber. This may be heard with a stethoscope. It is called a murmur.

Did you know that each wiggly line on a heart monitor is in relationship to the heart pumping blood through the heart? Changes in the wiggly line can tell health care providers which part of your heart is not working. The way the wiggly line looks can tell health care providers if the top part of the heart and or the bottom part of the heart is in distress. Go wiggly lines because no wiggly heart lines, are not cool!

Hard Restart-Strength to Weaknesses

A hard restart is overwhelming time in an individual's life. It takes great strength from within to avoid the crashing and overwhelming moments of life. Yet, once the individual gets a foot hold again, then life is a banquet of opportunities.

The individual will learn their weaknesses quickly. Much of this will become apparent. To move forward, the strengths need to become the focus. The strength of finding shelter, food, coping skills to deal with losses of family, friends, and work opportunities.

Focusing on the moments, daily and weekly strengths, will build confidences again. It will help increase the coping skills of the individual. The importance of this is that life is never just one line connected by two dots but more of a wild roller coaster with lots of ups, downs, flips, and just try and "keep the arms inside the ride" of life. The more the individual gains confidence, the less overwhelming the restart will be.

Hard Restart Deteriorating Health

A hard restart is when life happens and through no fault of your own, everything may come crashing apart. During all this time of change and chaos, the individual's health may take a toll that makes a hard restart nearly impossible to get through.

Mentally, it will be hard. The losses can be great and hard to deal with. Please reach out to your health care provider. There are options from a listening ear, counseling, and medications for short term use for anxiety and depression.

Physically, it is wise to get a checkup of the body systems. Chaotic changes can challenge the body's organs and cause health to deteriorate that may cause a need for vitamins, medications, or testing to discern if any intervention is needed by the health care provider.

Immunity may have also deteriorated and should be evaluated by a health care provider. Corrective intervention may include vitamins, vaccines, or medications, after testing and evaluation has been done. Do not let lack of insurance keep you from seeing a provider. There are many providers who provide concierge care, self-pay, free clinics, and many other options.

Hard Restart-Tiny X of Life

There is a time when life may come to an abrupt halt. It is called a hard restart. Life happens and through no fault of your own, everything may come crashing apart.

X--You are here. The tiny x on the map of life where you find yourself. Then what? By this point, the individual has begun the hard restart. Life has completely changed or changed enough that the prior life seems like a dream or life time ago. Time and life may have moved so fast that the individual's mind has been left on defense and not offense.

Then the time comes when the individual finally can go on the offense of life. Moving forward again. Establishing a new home, new friends and family, realizing that dreams and opportunities are possible, and that a new path has been laid out before them to follow or not.

Time. It will take time and the individual may not be quite ready for this undertaking or realize fully that the time invested may be longer than expected or available. It will be okay. Rome was not built in a day they say, but it sure did stand for a long time. As long as the individual stays persistent and moving forward, the hard restart will fade into the past as the new life becomes a reality. It is all good.
 The tiny x will move on the map of life.

Hard Restart-Emoticons of Feelings.

What is a Hard Restart?

Life happens and through no fault of your own, everything may come crashing apart. It could be a job loss. Loss of living arrangements. Parting ways in relationships. Even weather related events that leave individuals wondering what to do now?

Once the basics of shelter and food have been established. Where does one move on from this point? The sky can be the limit and it can be overwhelming.

First stop: emotions. The stages and emotions of grieving may begin. However, circumstances may not give the individual immediate access to allow emotions of grieving to commence. Individuals may have to power through life at the moment and put emotions on the side for later. It may come as a surprise to the individual, later when safety and life seems to improve, the emotions break. Go ahead and grieve. It is okay. Laugh out loud! It is okay. Cry your eyes out. It is okay. Represent all the emoticons of life. It is still okay. Just realize that if moving on is becoming too painful, reach out for help. It is okay. Sometimes we need help or just someone to listen. It is okay.

Second: accepting. Accepting what has happened does not mean it was fair, right, wrong, or anything other than acknowledging it happened. It just means that the individual has accepted their life has suddenly changed. Acknowledgment allows the individual to begin to work through where they are and where they may want to be. It may take some time. This is okay.

Hard Life Restart- The Basics.

Life happens and through no fault of your own, everything may come crashing apart. It could be a job loss. Loss of living arrangements. Parting ways in relationships. Even weather related events that leave individuals wondering what to do now?

Hard restarts are not easy. The basics are the first thing targeted. Where do I sleep tonight? Where do I get something to eat? Where can I store my items of importance I have left?

Housing: Shelters offer temporary housing and may be limited and restrictions. Family and friends may be willing to help out with temporary living conditions. Bed and breakfast, tents in parks, small camper/RV communities, and inexpensive hotels may offer options to those with monetary funds.

Food: It may not always be freely available in preference or dietary restrictions. Pantries offer free food but limit the time available or access with restrictions. Places of worship may offer free meals or have pantries to people in their communities. Government assistance with food may be obtain but paperwork and qualifications will be needed, such as physical address of residence, or emergency residence.

Storage: This can vary from leaving it behind, storing at friend or family, selling or donating, and finding reasonable storage units.

Each circumstance is individual and resources vary depending on individual. Restarting is hard but not impossible. Sometimes a hard restart gives an individual choices or opportunities not realized before a hard life restart.

Wicking Cold

There is a term called wicking. It references drawing water from one area to another via clothing or cloth. Wicking clothes can pull moisture away from the body and products exist on today's market for purchase.

Now let us think of wicking on a larger scale. Chairs, couches, beds, and like furniture. These items pushed up against a wall will help wick the cold from the walls and windows to the furniture. Persons resting in the furniture, will then wick the cold to them as well. This can cause the individual to become ill.

To prevent wicking cold and getting sick, pull all furniture away from walls. Especially baby cribs. Furniture pulled away approximately four inches will help prevent wicking cold and may prevent illness.

Freezing? Do Housework!

It is the time of year when it is starting to get colder than one can stand. Back in late October or early November, the furnace was turned on. Now it has gotten even colder. Turning up the heat will also mean emptying out the wallet of cold hard cash. What else could you do?

Plain and simple, housework.

1. Run the dishwasher. Leave the heat setting on.

2. Keep the laundry done up and the dryer running. There is nothing like warm towels and blankets at this time of year!

3. Heat up water on the stove. Moisture in the air helps heat the house.

These three easy tips will help heat up a home a few degrees without having to increase the thermostat for more heat.